Achieve Your Weight Loss Targets

A complete guide to a healthy you.

DAN OHTEE

Summary

"We'll take you on a life-changing journey through the realm of weight loss in "Achieve Your Weight Loss Targets" covering themes like:
- Recognizing your body composition and establishing reasonable objectives
- Meal planning and nutrition techniques for long-term weight loss
- Plans for physical activity and exercise to increase metabolism

- Overcoming setbacks and staying motivated
- Optimal weight loss through stress, sleep, and water management
- Sustaining weight loss over the long run and preventing plateaus This eBook's professional guidance, applicable examples, and helpful hints will enable you to:
- Give up fast fixes and fad diets.
- Establish a sensible and balanced relationship with diet and physical activity.

- Develop a resilient and
strong mindset
- Reach your weight loss goals
and stay at a healthy weight
for the rest of your life.

 Come along with us on this
path to a happy, healthier you.
Now let's get going!

TABLE OF CONTENTS

Summary

Introduction

PART ONE: UNDERSTANDING WEIGHT LOSS

Chapter 1: The Science behind Weight Loss

Chapter 2: Setting Realistic Goals and Expectations

CHAPTER 3: Recognizing the measurements and what your body is made of

Part 2: Nutrition and Weight Loss

CHAPTER 4: Macronutrients and Weight Loss (carbs, protein, fat)

Chapter 5: Micronutrients and Weight Loss (vitamins, minerals)

Chapter 6: Meal Planning and Portion Control

Part 3: Exercise and Weight Loss

Chapter 7: Exercise's Crucial Role in Losing Weight

Chapter 8: Cardiovascular Workouts and Loss of Weight.

Chapter 9: Resistance Training and Weight Loss

Chapter 10: High-Intensity Interval Training (HIIT) and Weight Loss

Part 4: Modifying Your Lifestyle to Lose Weight

Chapter 11: Reducing Stress and Losing Weights

Chapter 12: Losing Weight and Sleep

Chapter 13: Losing Weight and Hydration

Chapter 14: Social Support and Weight Loss:

Part 5: Overcoming Challenges and Maintaining Weight Loss

Chapter 15: Overcoming Plateaus and Weight Loss Plateaus

Chapter 16: Maintaining Weight Loss Long-Term

Chapter 17: Overcoming Obstacles and Relapsing in Weight Loss

Chapter 18: Creating a Positive Connection with Food and Activity

Conclusion

Introduction

"Welcome to Achieve Your Weight Loss Targets, a thorough and inspiring manual for accomplishing your weight reduction objectives and embracing a happier, healthier version of yourself. It takes more than just the numbers on the scale to lose weight—you also need to change the way you think about food, your body, and yourself. This eBook is intended to be your reliable travel companion, giving you a thorough understanding of the science underlying weight loss, doable tactics for long-term success, and the inspiration to get past setbacks and continue on course.

In these pages, you will find: – The science underlying macronutrients, micronutrients, and meal planning for optimal weight reduction

- The keys to creating
reasonable and attainable
weight loss objectives
- The value of physical activity
and exercise in increasing
metabolism and changing your
body
- Motivational thinking and
strategies to get past self-
doubt, cravings, and plateaus
- The importance of hydration,
sleep, and stress management
for weight loss and general
wellbeing
- Tried-and-true methods for
preventing relapses and

sustaining weight loss over
time

PART ONE:
UNDERSTANDING
WEIGHT LOSS

Chapter 1: The Science behind Weight Loss

In Wisconsin, almost one-third of people are obese. The science of weight loss and how to effectively shed pounds is a topic of constant study, which makes sense given the numerous health concerns and difficulties linked to obesity. Even though there are a plethora of diets and weight reduction regimens available, many people find it challenging to discover a weight loss approach that works and maintains the weight loss. Tammy Kindel, MD, PhD, a bariatric surgeon and associate professor at Froedtert and the Medical College of Wisconsin (MCW), discussed the science of weight loss, why it can be difficult to maintain weight loss, and how bariatric surgery can improve the lives of some patients in a recent Coffee Conversations with Scientists episode.

What Is Obesity and Why Is Your Health at Risk? In Wisconsin, sixty-five percent of people have a body mass index (BMI) of 25 to thirty or higher, meaning they are obese. Obesity is typically brought on by a person consuming more calories than they "burn" Obesity is also influenced by genetics, environment, and lifestyle factors. Why does obesity pose a health risk? It poses a risk for numerous grave illnesses and ailments, such as type 2 diabetes, infertility, elevated blood pressure, heart conditions, Cancers of the breast, colon, and endometrium fatty liver disease, gallbladder disease, stroke, elevated cholesterol breathing issues, including apnea during sleep persistent pain in the lower back, arthritic Regrettably, certain groups are more vulnerable than others to related health hazards. "People who are growing up in areas where there is a lot of community stress, low socioeconomic status, limited access to food resources, and inadequate nutrition education are undoubtedly more likely to gain weight and experience serious medical complications related to being overweight," stated Dr. Kindel. For obese patients to see improvements in their health, weight loss is imperative. The Centers for Disease Control and Prevention state that among other health advantages, losing just 5 to 10% of your body weight can help improve blood pressure, blood cholesterol, and blood sugar levels.

What Is the Science of Weight Loss? Eating less and burning more calories are the keys to losing weight, or maintaining a healthy body weight. The body goes into a calorie deficit, which results in weight reduction, when more calories are burned than are taken in. Despite the formula's apparent simplicity, a variety of factors affect how many calories we consume.

"Many mechanisms regulate food intake through signals, in

our brain and our periphery, that give us signs for hunger and satiety (feeling full)," says Dr. Kindel. In addition, our body controls the burn, or output, through our metabolic rate and the ways in which it is influenced by hormones, illnesses, and drugs. The science of weight loss involves more than just tracking calories in and calories out. You can lose weight and keep it off by focusing on regular, moderate physical exercise and making healthy dietary choices (such as increasing whole fruits and vegetables, cutting back on sugary drinks, and eliminating trans fats). Maintaining weight loss after reaching a weight loss goal is not always simple. Many people who lose a substantial amount of weight gain it back two or three years later. So why is maintaining weight reduction so difficult? People frequently alter their lifestyle, exercise routine, and food drastically in an attempt to reduce weight. This could entail exercising more frequently or in different ways, as well as reducing or eliminating specific food groups. But once the target weight is lost, keeping the weight off depends on keeping up the new habits and way of living. In the CCWS episode, Dr. Kindel talked about a research on weight, metabolism, and exercise that involved participants from the well-known reality TV program "The Biggest Loser," which focuses on weight loss. Researchers discovered that a large number of people who were successful in losing and maintaining their weight long after the show had a high metabolic adaptation, which means that even years after the competition, their metabolic rates had not returned to normal. This shows that by sticking to their diet and exercise plans from the competition, individuals were able to maintain their weight loss after appearing on the show.

Dr. Kindel stated that maintaining weight loss requires sticking to the dietary and exercise modifications adopted. Significant weight loss isn't always the result of willpower or cerebral cortex alone. Numerous signals are involved. Since we don't always have control over our metabolic rate, the study's main lesson for me as a physician is that "what gets you there (in a diet) stays you there." Who Can Get Bariatric Surgery and What Does It Entail? A weight-loss strategy called bariatric surgery involves shrinking the stomach, which can aid in consuming less food. Bariatric surgery is the best course of action for certain patients seeking long-term weight loss and improved health. Dr. Kindel explained that if you have a medical condition linked to obesity and your body mass index is between 30 and 35, you may be a candidate for bariatric surgery. Even if you haven't yet experienced one of those health issues, there is a cardiovascular risk reduction if your body mass index is 35 or above.

In this case, we believe that the danger of surgery is lower than the risk of long-term untreated obesity. The Roux-en-Y Gastric Bypass and Sleeve Gastrectomy are the two most popular bariatric procedures carried out at Froedtert and MCW. These procedures modify the body's signals regarding food intake, the amount of food required to feel full, and can lower hunger hormones. A patient's eligibility for bariatric surgery is determined by a number of factors, including their medical history, body mass index, and preferences. 38% of program participants, regardless of insurance status, report experiencing food insecurity, according to a survey done by researchers (not having enough or appropriate food for a healthy life). As a result, screening for food insecurity was made mandatory for all bariatric surgery patients in order to guarantee high-quality care for patients from all socioeconomic backgrounds. Patients in the program are required to follow a protein shake diet for two weeks prior to any bariatric surgery in order to decrease surgical risks and shrink the size of the liver. The Medical Weight Loss and Bariatric Surgery Program established a protein shake food bank where patients can donate and take home unopened and unused protein powders in order to assist every patient have access to and benefit from the shakes this procedure requires. Dr. Kindel offers these guidelines for weight maintenance, regardless of the diet plan you choose to follow:

Avoid consuming calories from juice, sugar-filled coffee drinks, alcohol, and other sources; monitor your eating and lifestyle to be more accountable; and Choose an enjoyable aerobic activity to maintain cardiovascular health, and then incorporate strength training to build muscle. The most crucial factor in choosing a weight loss plan that will work for you is being realistic about your lifestyle and the changes you

can honestly commit to
making.

Chapter 2: Setting Realistic Goals and Expectations

Weight loss is a journey that requires patience, dedication, and a clear understanding of what can be achieved. Setting realistic goals and expectations is crucial to this journey, as it helps individuals stay motivated, focused, and committed to their weight loss plan. In this essay, we will explore the importance of setting realistic goals and expectations in weight loss, and provide guidance on how to do so effectively.

The Importance of Realistic Goals

Setting realistic goals is essential in weight loss because it helps individuals avoid disappointment, frustration, and burnout. Unrealistic expectations can lead to a cycle of failure, where individuals become discouraged and give up on their weight loss efforts. Realistic goals, on the other hand, provide a sense of accomplishment and motivation, as individuals see progress and achievements along the way.

Moreover, realistic goals promote sustainable weight loss. When individuals aim for unrealistic weight loss targets, they often resort to unhealthy and unsustainable methods, such as extreme calorie restriction or fad diets. These methods may lead to short-term weight loss, but they are often ineffective and even harmful in the long term. Realistic goals, on the other hand, encourage individuals to adopt healthy and sustainable habits, such as balanced eating and regular exercise, which promote long-term weight loss and overall health.

How to Set Realistic Goals

So, how can individuals set realistic goals and expectations in weight loss? Here are some guidelines:

1. Consult with a healthcare professional or registered dietitian to determine a healthy weight range and create a personalized weight loss plan.

2. Set specific, measurable, achievable, relevant, and time-bound (SMART) goals. For example, "I want to lose 10 pounds in the next 3 months" is a more effective goal than "I want to lose weight."

3. Break down large goals into smaller, manageable

milestones. This helps to maintain motivation and track progress.

4. Focus on progress, not perfection. Weight loss is not always linear, and it's normal to experience setbacks. Don't get discouraged by minor

5. Be realistic about your timeline. Aim to lose 1-2 pounds per week for a sustainable weight loss.

6. Consider your lifestyle and habits. Don't set goals that

require drastic changes that are hard to maintain.

7. Focus on health, not just weight loss. Aim to improve overall health and well-being, rather than just reaching a certain number on the scale.

8. Celebrate small victories along the way. Recognize and celebrate progress, no matter how small.

9. Be kind to yourself. Remember that setbacks are

normal and don't define your entire journey.

10. Stay consistent and patient. Weight loss takes time, and it's important to stay committed to your goals.

By following these guidelines, individuals can set realistic goals and expectations in weight loss, promoting a healthy, sustainable, and successful journey. Remember, weight loss is not just about reaching a certain weight, but about adopting a healthy lifestyle that improves overall well-being. By setting realistic goals and focusing on progress, individuals can achieve a healthier, happier life.

CHAPTER 3: Recognizing the measurements and what your body is made of

Knowing your dimensions and body composition is crucial when starting a weight loss plan. This information aids in goal-setting, progress monitoring, and well-informed food and exercise choices. We'll explore the essential elements of body composition and measurements in this essay, giving you a thorough grasp of the steps involved in effective weight loss. What You Should Know About Body Composition? The ratios of the many parts that comprise your body are referred to as your body composition. These components include:

– Fat Mass (FM): Total body fat, including subcutaneous (under the skin) and visceral (around organs) fat. The quantity of non-fat tissue, such as muscle, bone, and water, is known as lean body mass (LBM).

- Water: The volume of water that varies throughout the day in your body.
- Bone Density: Your bones' strength and density.
Measuring: Comprehending the Figures It's critical to comprehend the various measurements and what they signify when monitoring progress:
- Weight: The total weight of the body, which might change as a result of muscular growth or water retention.
- Body Fat Percentage (BF%): The proportion of body fat,

which is a more reliable measure of development than weight alone.
– Waist Circumference (WC): Indicates health hazards by measuring the amount of fat around your midsection.
– Hip-to-Waist Ratio (HWR): Determines the percentage of fat in your waist and hips and highlights potential health concerns.
– Body Mass Index (BMI): Relatively accurate, but limited, measure of body fat based on height and weight.
Evaluating Your

Measurements and Body Composition You can evaluate your measurements and body composition in a number of methods, such as:
- DXA, or dual-energy X-ray absorptiometry
- Weighing hydrostatically
- Measurements of the skinfold The analysis of bioelectrical impedance (BIA) Scales of Body Fat. It's crucial to speak with a qualified dietician or healthcare provider to find the approach that works best for you.

It's also critical to comprehend the various body fat categories and the associated health risks:

- Essential fat: required for body functions; 10–13% for men and 16–19% for women. Sports fat (14–17% for men, 20–23% for women) is common among athletes and people with a lot of muscle mass.

- Fitness fat (18–21% for males and 24-27% for women): this is normal for those whose muscle and fat content is in a healthy range.

- Average fat: average for the general population, with men averaging 22-25% and women 28-31%.
- Obesity: linked to increased health risks: 26% or higher for males and 32% or higher for women.

When evaluating your dimensions and body composition, it's critical to take the following into account:
- Progress, not perfection: place more emphasis on modest, long-lasting

adjustments than on
significant, abrupt changes
- Consistency: Monitor your
development on a frequent
basis to guarantee accuracy
and inspiration
- Holistic approach: rather
than concentrating only on
weight loss, take into account
your general health and well-
being.

Knowing your measurements
and body composition will
allow you to:
- Establish reasonable
expectations and goals.

- Monitor your progress and maintain motivation
- Make wise choices regarding your diet and exercise regimen
- Enhance your general health and wellbeing Recall that losing weight is about developing a strong, healthy body that will serve you for years to come, not simply about the number on the scale.

To begin your journey, speak with a qualified nutritionist or healthcare expert right away!

Part 2: Nutrition and Weight Loss

CHAPTER 4: Macronutrients and Weight Loss (carbs, protein, fat)

Reducing calories is a common strategy for weight loss, but it often ignores the significance of maintaining a balance between macronutrients. Understanding the roles that the macronutrients—fat, protein, and carbs—play in weight loss can help people design a weight loss strategy that works for them.

Carbohydrates: The body's main source of energy, broken down into glucose to power cells and organs
- Critical for fiber intake, mental clarity, and bodily function.

The role of weight loss:
- Give you energy for exercise and daily tasks
- Assist in maintaining muscle mass

- Carbs high in fiber facilitate digestion and satiety.

Protein
- Helps maintain muscle mass after weight reduction
- Regulates hormones and the immune system
- Develops and repairs tissues, including muscle, bone, and skin.

The role of weight loss:
Maintains muscular mass, increasing metabolism;
Aids in controlling portion sizes and satisfaction;

Promotes optimal bone density.

Fat:
- Energy-producing and nutrient-absorbing;
- Necessary for immune system, hormone regulation, and brain function.
- Contains both good (unsaturated) and bad (saturated and trans) fats.

The role of weight loss:
- Promotes hormone function and long-term energy.

- Nutrient absorption and satiety are aided by healthy fats.
- A healthy inflammatory response is supported.

Macronutrient Balancing for Weight Loss:
- Take into account individual demands depending on age, gender, body composition, and activity level
- Aim for a balanced ratio: 45–65% carbohydrates, 15-20% protein, and 20–35% fat

- Put an emphasis on whole, unprocessed foods to ensure nutrient-dense intake.

A balanced macronutrient intake is essential for successful weight loss. Understanding the functions of fat, protein, and carbs helps people design a customized diet that meets their needs and encourages long-term weight loss. Recall that the secret to reaching and keeping a healthy weight is a balanced diet, frequent exercise, and good living practices.

It's critical to comprehend the functions of every macronutrient as well as the caliber of the foods you eat. Give priority to complete, unprocessed foods such as fruits, vegetables, whole grains, lean meats, and healthy fats. Steer clear of processed snacks, quick meals, and sugary drinks as these can impede your attempts to lose weight. Portion control is another essential component of a balanced macronutrient diet for weight loss. To keep your calorie intake in check, watch serving sizes and portion sizes. You can accomplish this by cutting back on the amount of food you eat overall or by eating smaller, more frequent meals throughout the day.

Finally, keep in mind that overall lifestyle behaviors play a significant role in weight loss in addition to the balance of macronutrients. For the purpose of reaching and keeping a healthy weight, regular exercise, stress reduction, and enough sleep are all essential.

To sum up, maintaining a balance between macronutrients is essential for weight loss. With knowledge of the functions of fat, protein, and carbs together with an emphasis on whole, unprocessed meals, portion management, and healthy living practices, people can design a customized weight loss program that works for them and encourages long-term weight loss.

Keep in mind that losing
weight involves more than just
reducing your caloric intake; it
also involves feeding your
body the correct meals and
lifestyle choices to promote
general health and wellbeing.

Chapter 5: Micronutrients and Weight Loss (vitamins, minerals)

When it comes to weight loss, many people focus on macronutrients like carbohydrates, protein, and fat, but neglect the importance of micronutrients like vitamins and minerals. Micronutrients play a crucial role in weight loss, as they help regulate metabolism, energy production, and nutrient absorption. In this essay, we'll explore the role of micronutrients in weight loss and how they can support a healthy weight loss journey.

Vitamins:

- Vitamin B12: plays a crucial role in energy production and metabolism
- Vitamin D: regulates appetite and satiety hormones
- Vitamin B6: helps with fat metabolism and energy production
- Folate: supports healthy cell growth and metabolism

Minerals:

- Iron: essential for healthy red blood cells and oxygen transport
- Zinc: supports immune function and protein synthesis
- Magnesium: regulates blood sugar and insulin sensitivity
- Potassium: helps with water balance and blood pressure regulation

Micronutrient Deficiencies and Weight Loss:

- Deficiencies can lead to slowed metabolism, fatigue, and increased hunger
- Can impair nutrient absorption and energy production
- May lead to overeating and poor food choices

Food Sources and Supplements:

- Whole foods like fruits, vegetables, whole grains, lean proteins, and healthy fats provide essential micronutrients

- Supplements can fill nutrient gaps, but should not replace a balanced diet

Micronutrients like vitamins and minerals play a vital role in weight loss by regulating metabolism, energy production, and nutrient absorption. Deficiencies can hinder weight loss efforts, while adequate intake can support a healthy weight loss journey. Focus on whole foods and consider supplements if necessary. Remember, a balanced diet and healthy lifestyle habits are key to achieving and maintaining a healthy weight.

In addition to supporting weight loss, micronutrients also play a crucial role in overall health and well-being. They help to:

- Boost immune function
- Support healthy skin, hair, and nails
- Maintain healthy bones and muscles
- Regulate blood sugar and insulin levels

- Support healthy digestion
and gut health

Deficiencies in micronutrients
can lead to a range of health
problems, including:

- Fatigue and weakness
- Poor wound healing
- Hair loss and skin problems
- Weakened immune system
- Poor digestion and gut health

Fortunately, ensuring
adequate intake of
micronutrients is relatively
easy. A balanced diet that

includes a variety of whole foods can provide all the necessary micronutrients. Some key food sources include:

- Leafy greens (vitamin B12, iron)
- Citrus fruits (vitamin C)
- Nuts and seeds (magnesium, zinc)
- Fatty fish (vitamin D)
- Whole grains (folate, potassium)

In addition to a balanced diet, supplements can also be

helpful in filling any nutrient gaps. However, it's important to consult with a healthcare professional before starting any supplements to ensure safety and effectiveness.

Micronutrients play a vital role in weight loss and overall health. Ensuring adequate intake through a balanced diet and supplements can support a healthy weight loss journey and overall well-being. Remember, a healthy weight loss journey is not just about cutting calories, but also about nourishing your body with the right foods and nutrients to support optimal health.

Furthermore, micronutrients can also play a role in reducing inflammation, which is a known risk factor for chronic diseases such as heart disease, diabetes, and certain cancers. Vitamins like vitamin C and E, as well as minerals like zinc and selenium, have anti-inflammatory properties that can help to reduce inflammation and promote overall health.

In addition, micronutrients can also support healthy gut bacteria, which is essential for a strong immune system and overall health. Vitamins like vitamin K and biotin, as well as minerals like calcium and magnesium, can help to support the growth of healthy gut bacteria.

Finally, micronutrients can also play a role in reducing stress and anxiety. Vitamins like vitamin B12 and minerals like magnesium and potassium can help to regulate the body's response to stress and promote relaxation.

In conclusion, micronutrients play a vital role in overall health and well-being, and can support weight loss, reduce inflammation, promote healthy gut bacteria, and reduce stress and anxiety. Ensuring adequate intake of micronutrients through a balanced diet and supplements can have a significant impact on overall health and well-being. It is important to

consult with a healthcare
professional to determine the
best course of action for
individual needs.

Chapter 6: Meal Planning and Portion Control

A balanced diet and weight management depend heavily on meal planning and quantity control. We can make sure we are obtaining the nutrients we need without overindulging and gaining weight by planning and regulating how much we eat. The advantages of meal planning and portion control will be discussed in this essay, along with suggestions for implementing these practices in day-to-day living.

The advantages of meal planning: Reduces food waste, promotes healthy eating, helps with weight management, and saves time and money.

The advantages of portion control Maintains a healthy weight; controls cravings and hunger; lessens the feeling of guilt associated with overindulging in food; and promotes general health and wellbeing.

Advice for Organizing Meals: Create a grocery list, plan your weekly meals, prepare ahead of time, and take your requirements and timetable into account.

Advice on Managing Portion Size: Make use of a food scale or measuring cups. Eat carefully and gently. Steer clear of eating in front of screens. Recognize serving sizes

One of the most effective strategies for developing good eating habits and managing weight is meal planning and portion control. These are daily behaviors that we might adopt to enhance our general health and wellbeing. Recall that the goal is to make deliberate decisions that support our bodies rather than starving ourselves. Plan ahead and manage your portions now to start on the path to a happy, healthier you!

Meal planning and portion management have additional advantages beyond those already discussed. They can assist with:
- Reducing worry and tension related to eating and food
- Cutting costs on eating out and groceries

- Improving gastrointestinal health and minimizing IBS symptoms
- Promoting general health and wellbeing, which includes lowering the chance of developing chronic illnesses like diabetes, heart disease, and some types of cancer.

 Try these suggestions to get started with portion control and meal planning:

- Use a meal planning app or website to help with ideas and organizing
- Measure out quantities using cups, scales, or your hands (e.g. a serving of protein is around the size of your palm)
- Start small and set reasonable objectives, such as planning one or two meals each day
- Savor your meal, eating slowly and deliberately, and observing your body's signals of hunger and fullness.

Treat yourself with kindness, and if you make a mistake, don't give up; just pick yourself up at the next meal. Recall that while portion management and meal planning are skills that require practice, the rewards are well worth the effort. You can enhance your relationship with food, lower your stress level, and improve your health by taking charge of your eating habits. A balanced diet and weight management depend heavily on meal planning and quantity control. We can make sure we are obtaining the nutrients we need without overindulging and gaining weight by planning and regulating how much we eat.

Anyone can start planning meals and controlling portion sizes and reaping the many advantages by using the advice provided in this essay. Meal preparation and portion management can also assist with:

By organizing meals around items that are already on hand, food waste can be decreased. Time can be saved by preparing meals ahead of time and having healthy options available. Mental health can be improved by lowering stress and anxiety related to food and eating.

Ensuring a varied and balanced diet to promote

general health and well-being. Try the following to develop meal planning and portion control as a long-lasting habit:

- Include others in the process, such as family or friends, to make it more fun and accountable
- Be flexible and allow for modifications in your plan if necessary
- Develop the habit of doing it every day
- Rejoice in little improvements and resist the

need to let losses depress you.

To sum up, meal planning and portion control are effective strategies for developing a balanced diet and controlling weight. We may enhance our general health and well-being, lessen stress and anxiety, and save time and money by organizing and regulating our food intake. We can make sure we eat a varied and balanced diet that

promotes our general health
and well-being by developing
the habit of being adaptable.
Recall that what matters is
not perfection but rather
development and making
well-informed decisions that
benefit our bodies and
minds.

Part 3: Exercise and Weight Loss

Chapter 7: Exercise's Crucial Role in Losing Weight

A key element of any weight loss program is exercise. Exercise is crucial for burning calories, gaining muscle, and speeding up metabolism—dieting and good eating practices are important, too.

Exercise's Advantages for Losing Weight:
Enhances insulin sensitivity and lowers the risk of chronic diseases;

-Builds muscle mass, which further raises metabolism;
-Burns calories and increases energy expenditure;
- Improves mood and mental health, lowering stress and anxiety
- Boosts motivation and responsibility.

Exercise Types for Losing Weight:
- Cardiovascular Aerobic Exercise: jogging, swimming, cycling, and brisk walking
- Resistance Training (also known as strength training):

bodyweight exercises, resistance bands, and weightlifting
- High-Intensity Interval Training (HIIT): quick bursts of vigorous activity interspersed with little rest intervals.

 Advice for Including Exercise in Your Daily Routine:
- Find an exercise partner or accountability buddy
- Start small, aiming for 150 minutes of moderate-intensity exercise each week
- Schedule exercise into your daily planner or calendar

- Vary your routine to prevent overuse injuries and plateaus
- Include physical exercise in routine duties, like walking or using the stairs to get to work.

A key element of any weight loss program is exercise. You may boost metabolism, gain muscle, and burn calories by include physical activity in your regular routine. To prevent hitting a plateau, always start small, locate a workout partner, and vary your regimen. Exercise can assist you in reaching your weight loss objectives and enhancing your general health and well-being with persistent effort and focus. Numerous psychological and emotional advantages of exercise might also help with weight loss.

Frequent exercise has been demonstrated to:
Diminish tension and unease
- Elevate happiness and general wellbeing
- Improve focus and cognitive performance
- Encourage higher-quality sleep

- Boost confidence in oneself and one's appearance

Exercise can also boost motivation and a sense of accomplishment, both of which are important components of maintaining a healthy weight. People can increase their likelihood of sticking to their weight reduction strategy by developing a good relationship with exercise and building confidence via the development and achievement of fitness goals.

To sum up, exercise is an essential part of any weight loss program. It has several psychological and emotional advantages that can help with weight loss in addition to burning calories and increasing muscle. Your chances of reaching and maintaining a healthy weight can be increased and your general health and well-being can be enhanced by adding regular physical activity to your daily routine. Always keep in mind that it's critical to discover a fitness regimen that you both enjoy and can fit into your lifestyle. Whichever physical activity you choose—walking, jogging, swimming, or weightlifting—the most crucial thing is to pick something you can commit to over time. When done consistently and with commitment, exercise can be an effective strategy for reaching and keeping a healthy weight.

Chapter 8: Cardiovascular Workouts and Loss of Weight.

Cardiovascular exercise, also known as aerobic exercise, is a crucial component of any weight loss plan. Regular cardio exercise not only burns calories and contributes to weight loss, but also provides numerous benefits for overall health and well-being. In this essay, we will explore the role of cardiovascular exercise in weight loss, its benefits, and provide tips on how to incorporate it into your daily routine.

Role of Cardiovascular Exercise in Weight Loss:

- Burns calories and increases energy expenditure
- Improves insulin sensitivity and reduces risk of chronic diseases
- Enhances mental health and mood, reducing stress and anxiety
- Increases motivation and accountability

Benefits of Cardiovascular Exercise:

- Improves heart health and reduces risk of heart disease
- Increases lung function and overall endurance
- Enhances muscle strength and tone
- Supports better sleep quality
- Boosts metabolism and burns fat

Types of Cardiovascular Exercise:

- Running

- Swimming
- Cycling
- Brisk walking
- Dancing
- High-Intensity Interval
Training (HIIT)

Tips for Incorporating
Cardiovascular Exercise into
Your Routine:

- Start small, aiming for 150
minutes of moderate-intensity
exercise per week
- Schedule exercise into your
daily planner or calendar

- Find an exercise buddy or accountability partner
- Mix up your routine to avoid plateaus and prevent overuse injuries
- Incorporate physical activity into daily tasks, such as taking the stairs or walking to work

Cardiovascular activity can also boost motivation and a sense of achievement, both of which are important factors in maintaining a healthy weight. People can increase their likelihood of sticking to their weight reduction strategy by developing a good relationship with exercise and building confidence via the development and achievement of fitness goals. Exercises that include the heart are essential to any weight loss program. It has several psychological and emotional advantages that can help with weight loss in addition to burning calories and enhancing general health. You can attain a healthy weight, boost motivation, and enhance your general health and well-being by adding frequent cardiac exercise to your daily regimen. Recall that it's critical to choose a cardiovascular fitness regimen that complements your lifestyle and that you love. The most crucial thing is to choose a long-term physical activity that you enjoy, whether it's swimming, cycling, dancing, or jogging. Cardiovascular exercise can be an effective tool for reaching and maintaining a healthy weight if done with perseverance and dedication.

Other benefits of cardiovascular exercise are numerous. As an illustration:
- Better cardiovascular health: Frequent cardiovascular activity lowers the risk of heart disease and improves circulation by strengthening the heart and lungs.
- Enhanced muscular strength and endurance: Cardiovascular activity helps enhance muscular strength and endurance, which facilitates daily tasks and lowers the chance of injury.

- Increased bone density: Cardio exercises that involve weight bearing, such jogging or leaping, can help increase bone density and lower the risk of osteoporosis and fractures.

- Better mental health: Research has indicated that engaging in cardiovascular exercise can improve mental health by lowering stress and anxiety levels and elevating mood. To sum up, cardiovascular activity is an essential part of living a healthy lifestyle. It can be tailored to accommodate a variety of interests and fitness levels and provides a host of advantages for both mental and physical health. You may raise your energy levels, lower your chance of developing chronic diseases, and enhance your general health and well-being by including regular cardiac exercise in your regimen.

So why not begin right now? Make regular cardiac exercise a part of your routine by finding an exercise you enjoy.

Both your body and mind will appreciate it! Never forget that you should always get medical advice before beginning a new fitness regimen, particularly if you have any underlying medical issues or concerns. They can assist you in figuring out which kind and level of cardiovascular exercise is ideal for your particular requirements and capacity.

Chapter 9: Resistance Training and Weight Loss

Resistance training, also known as strength training, is a crucial component of any weight loss plan. While cardiovascular exercise is essential for burning calories, resistance training builds muscle mass, which is vital for increasing metabolism and achieving sustainable weight loss. In this essay, we will explore the role of resistance training in weight loss, its benefits, and provide tips on how to incorporate it into your daily routine.

Role of Resistance Training in Weight Loss:

- Builds muscle mass, increasing metabolism and burning more calories at rest
- Enhances muscle tone and strength, improving overall physical function
- Increases bone density, reducing the risk of osteoporosis and fractures

- Improves insulin sensitivity, reducing the risk of chronic diseases

Benefits of Resistance Training:

- Increases muscle mass and strength
- Improves bone density
- Enhances metabolic rate
- Improves insulin sensitivity
- Supports better sleep quality
- Boosts self-esteem and body confidence

Types of Resistance Training:

- Free weights (dumbbells, barbells)
- Resistance bands
- Machines (leg press, chest press)
- Bodyweight exercises (push-ups, squats)

Tips for Incorporating Resistance Training into Your Routine:

- Start with 2-3 times per week and gradually increase frequency

- Focus on compound exercises (squats, deadlifts, bench press)
- Use progressive overload (increase weight or reps over time)
- Incorporate variety to avoid plateaus
- Seek guidance from a personal trainer or fitness professional

Resistance training is a vital component of any weight loss plan, building muscle mass and increasing metabolism. By incorporating resistance training into your daily routine, you can achieve sustainable weight loss, improve overall health, and enhance physical function. Remember to start slowly, focus on compound exercises, and seek guidance from a fitness professional. With consistent effort and dedication, resistance training can be a powerful tool in achieving your weight loss goals.

Resistance training also has numerous mental and

emotional benefits that can aid in weight loss. Lifting weights and doing resistance exercises can:

- Reduce stress and anxiety
- Improve mood and overall sense of well-being
- Enhance cognitive function and concentration
- Promote better sleep quality
- Increase self-esteem and body confidence

Furthermore, resistance training can also provide a sense of accomplishment and motivation, which can be a powerful tool in maintaining a healthy weight. By setting and achieving fitness goals, individuals can build confidence and develop a positive relationship with exercise, making it more likely that they will stick to their weight loss plan.

In conclusion, resistance training is a crucial component of any weight loss plan. It builds muscle mass, increases metabolism, and provides numerous physical and mental benefits. By incorporating resistance training into your daily routine, you can achieve sustainable weight loss, improve overall health, and enhance physical function. Remember to start slowly, focus on compound exercises, and seek guidance from a fitness professional. With consistent effort and dedication, resistance training can be a powerful tool in achieving your weight loss goals.

Chapter 10: High-Intensity Interval Training (HIIT) and Weight Loss

High-Intensity Interval Training (HIIT) has become a popular and effective way to achieve weight loss and improve overall health. HIIT involves short bursts of high-intensity exercise followed by brief periods of rest or low-intensity exercise. This type of training has been shown to be highly effective for burning calories, improving cardiovascular health, and increasing muscle strength.

Benefits of HIIT for Weight Loss:

- Time-Efficient: HIIT workouts are typically shorter than traditional cardio workouts, lasting anywhere from 15-30 minutes.
- Caloric Burn: HIIT workouts burn a high number of

calories, both during and after exercise.

- Improved Insulin Sensitivity: HIIT improves insulin sensitivity, reducing the risk of developing type 2 diabetes.

- Increased Muscle Strength: HIIT builds muscle strength and endurance.

- Improved Cardiovascular Health: HIIT improves cardiovascular health by increasing heart rate and blood flow.

Types of HIIT Workouts:

- Sprint Intervals: Short sprints followed by walking or jogging.
- Burpees: A full-body exercise that involves a squat, push-up, and jump.
- Tabata: 20 seconds of all-out effort followed by 10 seconds of rest.
- Kettlebell Swings: High-intensity swings using a kettlebell.

Tips for Incorporating HIIT into Your Routine:

- Start Slow: Begin with shorter intervals and gradually increase duration and intensity.
- Warm Up and Cool Down: Always warm up before starting a HIIT workout and cool down afterwards.
- Listen to Your Body: Rest when needed and don't push yourself too hard.
- Mix it Up: Vary your HIIT workouts to avoid plateaus.

High-Intensity Interval Training (HIIT) is a powerful tool for weight loss and overall health. Its time-efficient, caloric-burning, and muscle-building benefits make it an ideal workout for those looking to achieve weight loss and improve their health. By incorporating HIIT into your routine, you can achieve sustainable weight loss, improve cardiovascular health, and increase muscle strength. Remember to start slowly, listen to your body, and mix up your workouts to get the most out of HIIT.

Part 4: Modifying Your Lifestyle to Lose Weight

Chapter 11: Reducing Stress and Losing Weights

There is a close relationship between stress and weight reduction; persistent stress may impede attempts to lose weight and even cause weight gain. Our bodies release the hormone cortisol in response to stress, which encourages the storage of fat, especially around the middle. Stress can also result in emotional eating, bad food choices, and a lack of desire to exercise, all of which can impede attempts to lose weight.

Stress's Effect on Losing Weight:

- Cortisol production: Stress causes the release of cortisol, which increases the storage of fat and causes weight gain.

- Emotional eating: Stress can contribute to overindulgence, poor food selections, and emotional eating.

- Decreased motivation: Stress can make it harder to be

physically active, which can impede weight loss attempts.
 - Restless nights: Stress can throw off sleep cycles, which can result in weariness, hunger pangs, and weight gain.

Techniques for Stress Reduction That Work for Losing Weight:
- Mindfulness and meditation: Consistent mindfulness training lowers cortisol and stress levels.
 - Deep breathing exercises: By calming the body and mind,

deep breathing helps lower stress.

- Yoga and tai chi: These forms of exercise combine mindfulness with physical movement to ease tension and encourage relaxation.

- Journaling: Putting ideas and feelings on paper can aid in stress management and release.

- Social support: Establishing a robust support system can aid in stress management and encourage weight loss.

Extra Advice on Stress Management and Encouraging Weight Loss:

- Make sleep a priority. To control hunger hormones and aid with weight loss, aim for 7-9 hours of sleep per night.

- Get regular exercise: Exercise helps you lose weight and reduce stress and anxiety.

- Take care of yourself: Schedule leisure time for enjoyable and calming pursuits like reading or listening to music.

- Seek professional assistance: If stress and weight loss are recurring problems, think about getting advice from a certified dietician or mental health specialist.

Chronic stress can impede efforts and lead to weight gain, thus managing stress is essential to losing weight. Through the integration of efficacious stress management methodologies, such as mindfulness, deep breathing, and social support, individuals can mitigate stress, foster relaxation, and establish a more favorable milieu for weight reduction.

Recall that achieving a healthy lifestyle involves more than just making bodily adjustments—it also entails attending to the mental and emotional parts of it. Apart from the previously discussed stress management methods, there are various other approaches that may facilitate weight loss. Creating a calorie deficit—eating less calories than the body burns—is one of the best strategies for weight loss. Reducing daily calorie intake and increasing physical exercise can be combined to achieve this.

Eating a diet rich in nutrients is another crucial component of weight reduction. Make a point of eating entire, unprocessed foods such as fruits, vegetables, whole grains, and lean meats. Steer clear of processed snacks, sugar-filled beverages, and fast food that are heavy in empty calories and lacking in nutrients. Maintaining hydration is also essential for losing weight. Increased metabolism, better digestion, and appetite suppression can all be achieved by drinking lots of water. Try to consume eight glasses of water or more each day. Sleep is a critical component in weight loss. Sleep deprivation can mess with appetite hormones, causing binge eating and weight gain. Try to get seven to nine hours each night. Reducing stress is essential to losing weight. Through the integration of stress-reduction strategies such as mindfulness, deep breathing, and social support, people can establish a more favorable atmosphere for weight loss. Weight loss efforts can also be supported by maintaining a calorie deficit, eating meals high in nutrients, drinking enough of water, and getting adequate sleep.

Recall that losing weight is a journey that calls for endurance, patience, and a comprehensive strategy. People can live better, happier lives by addressing the psychological, emotional, and physical components of weight loss. There are numerous additional strategies to reduce stress and encourage weight loss. Including exercise in your daily routine is one practical strategy. Exercise releases endorphins, or "feel-good" hormones, which not only burn calories and aid in weight loss but also lessen tension and anxiety. Mindful eating is an additional method of stress management and weight reduction encouragement. This entails observing your body's signals of hunger and fullness, eating mindfully and slowly, and refraining from emotional eating. You may lessen stress-related eating and cultivate a better relationship with food by practicing mindful eating.

Moreover, managing stress and losing weight depend on obtaining adequate sleep. Sleep deprivation can mess with appetite hormones, causing binge eating and weight gain. To enhance the quality of your sleep, set up a calming nighttime routine and aim for 7-9 hours of sleep each night. Ultimately, getting social support from loved ones, friends, or a therapist can help you stay motivated and stress-free while trying to lose weight. When faced with obstacles, having a support system can offer emotional support, accountability, and encouragement.

In summary, controlling stress is essential to attaining and sustaining weight loss. Through the integration of stress-reduction strategies such as mindfulness, deep breathing, and social support, people can establish a more favorable atmosphere for weight loss. Moreover, maintaining an active lifestyle, obtaining enough sleep, and engaging in mindful eating can help with weight loss. Recall that losing weight is a journey that calls for endurance, patience, and a comprehensive strategy. People can live better, happier lives by addressing the psychological, emotional, and physical components of weight loss.

Chapter 12: Losing Weight and Sleep

Sleep has a major influence on weight loss and is essential for general health and wellbeing. Studies have repeatedly demonstrated that getting enough sleep can assist and even improve weight loss while sleep deprivation can undermine attempts to lose weight. This essay will examine the relationship between sleep and weight reduction and go over the

various ways that sleep
influences weight loss.

Sleep's Effect on Losing
Weight:
- Hormone Regulation: Leptin
and ghrelin, two hormones
that are linked to appetite, are
regulated by sleep. Lack of
sleep causes ghrelin levels to
rise, which increases hunger,
and leptin levels to fall, which
lessens feelings of fullness.
- Metabolism: Lack of sleep
slows down metabolic rate,
which makes it more difficult
to lose weight.

Sleep has an impact on metabolism.

- Cortisol: Lack of sleep raises cortisol levels, which promote the accumulation of belly fat.

- Insulin Sensitivity: Lack of sleep lowers insulin sensitivity, which can result in weight gain. Sleep has an impact on insulin sensitivity.

Advice for Boosting Weight Loss and Increasing Sleep Quality: Get morning sunlight exposure.

- Establish a regular sleep
schedule.
- Develop a soothing bedtime
routine.
- Optimize the sleep
environment (dark, quiet,
cool).
- Avoid stimulants before
bedtime.
- Avoid screens before
bedtime.

Neglecting sleep might make
weight loss efforts more
difficult. Sleep is a crucial
component of weight loss.

People can assist their weight loss efforts and enhance their general health by making sleep a priority and developing appropriate sleep habits. Sleep is not only a luxury—it is essential for general health. Keep this in mind. Sleep is also critical for muscle growth and recuperation, both of which are necessary for weight loss. Our muscles deteriorate during exercise, and they regenerate and mend while we sleep. We gain lean muscle mass through this process, which raises our metabolism and increases calorie burn even when we're at rest. Moreover, sleep has an impact on our mental well-being and willpower, both of which are essential for maintaining a weight loss program. Insufficient sleep can exacerbate stress, worry, and despair, which makes it more difficult to avoid bad meals and maintain our objectives.

Lastly, there is a connection between gut health and weight loss and how well we sleep. Lack of sleep has been linked

to altered gut microbial
balance, altered metabolism,
and altered appetite.

 In summary, sleep is an
essential part of losing weight,
and skipping it might make
things harder. We may boost
our chances of success,
enhance our general health,
and assist our weight
reduction journey by making
sleep a priority and developing
appropriate sleep habits.

Recall that getting enough
sleep is essential to reaching

our weight loss objectives
rather than just a luxury.

Chapter 13: Losing Weight and Hydration

Hydration has a major impact on weight loss and is essential for general health and wellbeing. While being dehydrated might impede weight loss efforts, staying properly hydrated can help. This essay will investigate the relationship between hydration and weight loss and go over the various ways that hydration influences weight reduction.

Hydration's Effect on Weight Loss:

- Accelerates Metabolism: Drinking enough water speeds up metabolism, which makes it easier for the body to burn calories.
- Suppresses Appetite: Consuming water helps lessen calorie intake and appetite.
- Enhances Digestion: Water aids in the breakdown of soluble fiber and nutrients,

increasing the body's ability to absorb them.

– Improves Exercise Performance: Staying properly hydrated makes workouts more efficient by improving physical performance.

– Decreases Water Retention: Drinking water helps decrease water retention, which promotes weight loss.

Advice on Appropriate Hydration and Losing Weight: Eat hydrating foods like watermelon, cucumbers, and celery; drink at least 8 cups (64

oz) of water every day; and stay away from dehydrating drinks like alcohol and caffeine.
- Watch the color and output of your urine;
- Hydrate before meals and when you exercise. Ignoring the importance of hydration in weight loss can impede results. Making proper hydration a priority and developing good drinking practices can help people lose weight and enhance their general health. Recall that maintaining adequate

hydration is essential to reaching your weight loss objectives.

Furthermore, drinking plenty of water can aid in lowering inflammation levels in the body, which is linked to metabolic disorders and obesity. In addition to decreasing the visibility of fine lines and wrinkles, drinking adequate water can make the skin look younger and more vibrant.

Additionally, drinking enough of water will enhance concentration and cognitive function, which will make it simpler to follow a diet and lead a healthy lifestyle. The symptoms of even minor dehydration, such as headaches, weariness, and difficulty concentrating, can make it more difficult to stick to a weight loss plan. Stress and worry are significant causes of overeating and making bad dietary decisions; drinking water can help lessen these feelings. Water consumption can help relax the body and mind, which lowers the risk of emotional eating and fosters a better connection with food. Achieving and maintaining a healthy weight depends on being hydrated, which is a key component of weight loss. Individuals can support their weight reduction journey, enhance their general health, and lead happier, healthier lives by emphasizing hydration and water intake. Beyond its physiological advantages, adequate water consumption can also improve mental well-being. Fatigue, anxiety, and despair are a few signs of dehydration that can make it more difficult to follow a weight reduction strategy. People who drink enough water can feel happier and experience less stress, which makes it simpler for them to make healthy decisions and maintain motivation while trying to lose weight. Moreover, staying hydrated might help with general appetite regulation and lessen cravings for unhealthy snacks.

Sometimes thirst can pass for hunger, which might result in overindulging or making bad dietary decisions. People can lessen their chance of overeating and make better decisions if they drink water throughout the day. Last but not least, being hydrated is crucial for both exercising and recovering. Maintaining adequate hydration can enhance strength, flexibility, and endurance, which will make it simpler to maximize training and achieve desired outcomes.

Furthermore, staying hydrated will shorten recovery times and lessen muscular discomfort, which will make it simpler to maintain a regular workout schedule.

In summary, staying hydrated is crucial to losing weight, and maintaining a healthy weight requires consuming adequate water. A happier, healthier life can be attained, weight reduction success can be increased, and general health can be improved by emphasizing hydration and water intake.

Recall that maintaining adequate hydration is an easy and efficient strategy to help with weight loss and enhance general health. People can raise their energy levels, decrease hunger and cravings, and speed up their metabolism by consuming eight glasses of water or more each day. Thus, pick up a bottle of water and begin drinking your way to a happier, healthier self!

Chapter 14: Social Support and Weight Loss:

Social support is a vital component of weight loss, providing motivation, encouragement, and accountability. Having a strong support system can make all the difference in achieving and maintaining weight loss goals. In this essay, we will explore the ways in which social support impacts weight loss and provide tips for cultivating a supportive network.

The Impact of Social Support
on Weight Loss:

- Emotional Support: Social
support provides emotional
encouragement, helping
individuals stay motivated and
focused on their weight loss
journey.
- Accountability: Social
support holds individuals
accountable for their actions,
reducing the likelihood of
slipping up or giving up.

- Shared Experience: Sharing
the weight loss journey with

others creates a sense of camaraderie and shared experience.

- Healthy Habits: Social support promotes healthy habits, such as regular exercise and healthy eating.

- Stress Reduction: Social support reduces stress levels, which can lead to overeating and weight gain.

Tips for Cultivating Social Support:

- Join a Weight Loss Group: Connect with others who share similar goals and experiences.

- Share Your Journey: Open up to friends and family about your weight loss journey.
- Find a Workout Buddy: Exercise with a friend or family member for motivation and accountability.

- Online Communities: Join online forums or social media groups for weight loss support.

- Supportive Partners: Involve your partner or spouse in your weight loss journey for added support.

Social support is a crucial element in achieving and maintaining weight loss. By surrounding yourself with a supportive network, you can stay motivated, accountable, and focused on your goals. Remember, weight loss is not just about physical changes, but also about emotional and mental well-being. Cultivate social support and watch your weight loss journey flourish! Additionally, social support can provide a sense of belonging and connection, which is essential for our overall well-being. When we feel supported and encouraged by others, we are more likely to stay committed to our weight loss goals and make healthy lifestyle choices. Moreover, social support can also help us develop a growth mindset, which is critical for weight loss success. When we surround ourselves with positive and supportive people, we are more likely to believe in ourselves and our ability to achieve our goals. Furthermore, social support can also provide a sense of accountability, which is crucial for weight loss. When we know that others are checking in on us and supporting us, we are more likely to stay on track and avoid slipping up.

Finally, social support can also help us celebrate our successes and milestones along the way, which is essential for staying motivated and encouraged. When we share our achievements with others, we are more likely to feel proud of ourselves and stay committed to our goals.

In conclusion, social support is a powerful tool for weight loss success. By surrounding ourselves with positive, supportive, and encouraging people, we can stay motivated, accountable, and focused on our goals. Remember, weight loss is not just about physical changes, but also about emotional and mental well-being. Cultivate social support and watch your weight loss journey flourish!

Part 5: Overcoming Challenges and Maintaining Weight Loss

Chapter 15: Overcoming Plateaus and Weight Loss Plateaus

Reaching a plateau is a common experience for individuals on a weight loss journey. Despite consistent effort and dedication, progress comes to a standstill, leaving individuals feeling frustrated and demotivated. However, plateaus are a normal part of the weight loss process, and there are strategies to overcome them.

Understanding Plateaus:

A plateau occurs when the body adapts to the current weight loss plan, making it less effective. This can happen due to various reasons such as:

- Metabolic adaptation
- Hormonal changes
- Loss of muscle mass
- Increased stress

Strategies to Overcome
Plateaus:

1. Reassess and Adjust:
    - Evaluate your current diet
and exercise plan
    - Identify areas for
modification
    - Make changes to shock
your body and stimulate
progress
2. Increase Intensity and
Duration:
    - Boost the intensity of your
workouts
    - Extend the duration of
your exercise sessions

- Challenge your body to
work harder
3. Change Your Exercise
Routine:
- Try new exercises or
activities
- Incorporate strength
training or high-intensity
interval training (HIIT)
- Keep your body guessing
4. Monitor Progress:
- Track your progress
through measurements,
weight, or body fat percentage
- Use a food diary or mobile
app to monitor your diet
- Stay accountable

5. Seek Support:

   - Share your struggles with a friend or family member

   - Join a weight loss support group

   - Consult with a healthcare professional or registered dietitian

6. Stay Hydrated and Get Enough Sleep:

   - Drink plenty of water throughout the day

   - Aim for 7-9 hours of sleep per night

   - Help your body recover and function optimally

7. Be Patient and Persistent:

- Weight loss is not always linear
- Plateaus are temporary
- Stay committed and focused

Overcoming plateaus requires patience, persistence, and strategic adjustments. By reassessing and adjusting your weight loss plan, increasing intensity and duration, changing your exercise routine, monitoring progress, seeking support, staying hydrated and getting enough sleep, and being patient and persistent, you can break through the plateau and continue your weight loss journey. Remember, weight loss is a journey, and plateaus are an opportunity to reassess and refine your approach. Stay committed, and you will achieve your weight loss goals.

Additionally, it's important to note that plateaus can be a sign of progress. When our bodies adapt to our weight loss efforts, it means that we've made significant changes and our bodies are responding. It's a sign that we're on the right track, and with a few adjustments, we can continue to make progress.

Another important aspect of overcoming plateaus is to focus on non-scale victories (NSVs). NSVs are measures of success that aren't necessarily reflected on the scale, such as increased energy levels, improved mood, or better sleep quality. By focusing on NSVs, we can see that we're making progress even if the scale isn't budging.

Finally, it's essential to remember that weight loss is not always linear. It's normal for progress to slow down or even stall at times. But with patience, persistence, and the right strategies, we can overcome plateaus and continue our weight loss journey.

In conclusion, plateaus are a normal part of the weight loss process, but they don't have to be a roadblock to success. By understanding the reasons for plateaus, reassessing and adjusting our weight loss plans, seeking support, and focusing on non-scale victories, we can overcome plateaus and achieve our weight loss goals. Remember, weight loss is a journey, and plateaus are just a bump in the road. Stay committed, and you will reach your destination.

Chapter 16: Maintaining Weight Loss Long-Term

Losing weight is a significant achievement, but maintaining weight loss long-term is an even greater challenge. Research shows that up to 80% of individuals who lose weight regain it within a year. However, with the right strategies and mindset, it is possible to maintain weight loss long-term.

Understanding the Challenges:

- Metabolic changes
- Hormonal fluctuations
- Increased appetite
- Social pressures

Strategies for Maintaining Weight Loss:

1. Healthy Eating Habits:
    - Balanced diet
    - Portion control
    - Mindful eating
2. Regular Physical Activity:
    - Aerobic exercise
    - Strength training

- High-intensity interval
training (HIIT)
3. Monitoring Progress:
   - Regular weigh-ins
   - Tracking food intake
   - Measuring body fat
percentage
4. Emotional Well-being:
   - Stress management
   - Self-care
   - Mindfulness practices
5. Social Support:
   - Weight loss support
groups
   - Online communities
   - Friends and family support
6. Continuous Learning:

- Nutrition education
- Fitness training
- Staying updated on latest research

Maintaining weight loss long-term requires a combination of healthy habits, emotional well-being, social support, and continuous learning. By understanding the challenges and implementing these strategies, individuals can increase their chances of successful long-term weight loss maintenance. Remember, weight loss is a journey, and maintenance is an ongoing process. Stay committed, and you will achieve long-term success.

Additionally, it's essential to focus on sustainable lifestyle changes rather than quick fixes or fad diets. This means adopting a balanced diet that includes a variety of whole foods, such as fruits, vegetables, whole grains, lean proteins, and healthy fats. It also means incorporating regular physical activity into your daily routine, such as walking, running, swimming, or weight training.

Another critical aspect of maintaining weight loss is staying hydrated. Drinking plenty of water throughout the day can help suppress appetite, boost metabolism, and support overall health. Aim for at least eight cups (64 ounces) of water per day.

Getting enough sleep is also crucial for weight loss maintenance. Aim for 7-9 hours of sleep per night to help regulate hunger hormones, support metabolism, and reduce stress.

Finally, it's important to be patient and persistent. Maintaining weight loss is a long-term process, and it's normal to experience setbacks or plateaus along the way. Don't get discouraged if you encounter obstacles – instead, focus on making progress, not perfection.

In conclusion, maintaining weight loss long-term requires

a combination of healthy habits, sustainable lifestyle changes, and ongoing support. By focusing on balanced eating, regular physical activity, staying hydrated, getting enough sleep, and being patient and persistent, individuals can increase their chances of successful weight loss maintenance. Remember, weight loss is a journey, and maintenance is an ongoing process. Stay committed, and you will achieve long-term success.

Chapter 17: Overcoming Obstacles and Relapsing in Weight Loss

Relapses and setbacks are unavoidable during the weight loss process. Even with the best of intentions, we could run into roadblocks that stop us in our tracks and leave us feeling disappointed, guilty, and frustrated. But it's important to keep in mind that obstacles are transient and may be surmounted with the appropriate attitude and techniques.

Recognizing Relapses and Setbacks: Relapses and setbacks can happen for a number of causes, including:
- Emotional consumption of food
- Insufficient drive
- Illness or injury Vacations or travel
- Constraints from society.

Techniques for Handling Failure and Recurrence:
1. Acknowledge and Accept:

- Identify the failure or relapse
- Take ownership of the situation
- Refrain from assigning blame or denying it

2. Determine Triggers:
- Consider the events that preceded the setback
- Recognize trends or causes
- Create coping mechanisms for triggers

3. Re-establish Your Course:
- Get back into a healthy eating routine

- Begin your workout regimen
again;
- Increase the duration and
intensity gradually

4. Seek Support:
- Talk to friends, relatives, or
medical professionals about
your challenges;
- Join a support group for
people trying to lose weight;
- Think about getting
professional assistance.

5. Develop Self-Compassion:
- Be kind and understanding
to yourself;

- Refrain from self-criticism
and negative self-talk;
- Put progress before of
perfection

6. Take A Lesson from the
Event:
- Consider what went wrong
- Determine what has to be
improved
- Create plans to avoid similar
mistakes in the future.

Relapses and setbacks are
common during the weight
loss process. We may
overcome challenges and carry

on with our weight loss quest by embracing setbacks, recognizing triggers, getting back on track, getting help, exercising self-compassion, and learning from the experience. Losing weight is a process rather than a goal. If you remain dedicated, you'll succeed in your endeavors.

It's also critical to concentrate on advancement rather than perfection. Reversals and setbacks are not signs of failure, but rather chances to improve and learn. We may cultivate resilience and persistence—two traits necessary for long-term weight loss success—by embracing a growth mindset. Self-care is another essential component in managing failures and relapses. Prioritizing our mental and physical health is essential, particularly in trying times. Take part in joyful and calming pursuits like yoga, meditation, or hobbies. Treat yourself with care and self-compassion, just as you would a close friend.

Recall that losing weight is a team effort. Seek for assistance from close friends and family, medical professionals, or online forums. Talking to people about your challenges and victories can be a great way to inspire and motivate yourself. Relapses and setbacks are unavoidable during the weight loss process. We may, however, overcome challenges and succeed in long-term weight reduction by embracing and admitting them, recognizing triggers, getting back on track, receiving help, engaging in self-compassion exercises, and concentrating on progress rather than perfection.

Recall that losing weight is a process rather than a goal. You will succeed if you remain dedicated to your goals.

Chapter 18: Creating a Positive Connection with Food and Activity

Developing a Positive Relationship with Food and Exercise: A Path to Wellbeing For general wellbeing, cultivating a positive relationship with diet and exercise is crucial. But in today's world, sedentary lifestyles, fad diets, and unattainable beauty standards frequently make this partnership difficult. In order to cultivate a positive connection with food and exercise, self-care, sustainability, and balance are crucial.

Food: Not an Obsession, but Nourishment. Consume a diet that is well-balanced, emphasizing whole, unprocessed foods such as vegetables, fruits, whole grains, lean meats, and healthy fats.
- Eat mindfully: Take pleasure in your food, observe your body's signals of hunger and

fullness, and eat without distractions. Get rid of the diet mentality by emphasizing progress over perfection and giving yourself the odd pleasure.

Exercise: Movement Rather Than Penalties
- Discover delight in movement: Whether it's dancing, weightlifting, or strolling, partake in physical activities that make you happy.
- Strive for consistency: Rather of overexerting oneself and running the risk of

burnout, aim for regular, moderate exercise.

- Pay attention to your body's needs. Give yourself time to heal and take care of yourself. It takes time, patience, and self-compassion to develop a positive relationship with food and exercise. You can develop a good and long-lasting approach to wellbeing by emphasizing nourishing foods, mindful eating, and happy movement.

Recall that progress, not perfection, is what matters.

Accept your path and acknowledge your little accomplishments along the road. It's also critical to understand that developing a positive connection with food and exercise is a process rather than a final goal.

The development of enduring habits and an optimistic outlook requires time, patience, and work. People can develop better eating and exercise habits by emphasizing progress rather than perfection.

Moreover, when developing a positive relationship with food and exercise, it's critical to give self-care and self-compassion first priority. This entails treating oneself with compassion and understanding as opposed to criticism or judgment. People can develop a positive and empowering perspective and lessen their stress and anxiety associated with food and exercise by engaging in self-care and self-compassion practices.

Ultimately, it's critical to understand that developing a positive connection with food and exercise is a shared experience. Seeking assistance from close friends and family, medical experts, or qualified dietitians can provide them the direction and motivation they require to achieve. Joining a community or group that prioritizes fitness and a healthy diet can also give you a sense of accountability and connection.

In conclusion, developing a positive connection with food and physical activity necessitates a holistic strategy that places an emphasis on self-care, self-compassion, happy movement, mindful eating, and nourishing. Individuals can develop a good and long-lasting approach to wellbeing by emphasizing progress rather than perfection and asking for help when they need it. Recall that developing a positive connection with food and exercise is a process rather

than a final goal. Accept your
path and acknowledge your
little accomplishments along
the road.

Conclusion

To sum up developing a positive connection with food and exercise is a journey that can be both empowering and transforming. A balanced and sustainable approach, along with letting go of cultural constraints, can help people build a good body image, enhance their physical and emotional well-being, and have a greater appreciation for activity and eating.

Recall that finding wellness is a journey rather than a destination. It is a voyage of self-love, self-discovery, and self-care. People can overcome the limitations of cultural expectations and embrace their own beauty, power, and perseverance by accepting this path. We urge you to continue on your own path towards developing a positive connection with food and fitness as we draw to a close this article. Begin with tiny adjustments, such as increasing the amount of nutritious foods in your diet or engaging in a joyful physical activity. Honor your accomplishments, no matter how modest, and treat yourself with kindness when you experience failures.

Above all, keep in mind that you are not traveling alone. Assemble a strong support system around you, consult medical professionals for advice, and make connections with like-minded others. Let's reinterpret what it means to be well and healthy together.

Let's cultivate an inclusive, accepting, and self-loving culture. And let's honor the diversity and beauty of the human experience in all of its guises. We appreciate you coming along for the ride. We hope that you will be able to establish a positive relationship with food and fitness.